kidney disease diet cookbook for women

Table of Contents:

Chapter 1
Introduction

Kidney disease, also known as chronic kidney disease (CKD), is a condition in which the kidneys gradually lose their ability to filter waste and excess fluids from the blood. This can lead to the accumulation of harmful substances in the body, which can have serious health implications. CKD is often a silent condition in its early stages, meaning many individuals may not realize they have it until significant damage has occurred. This makes awareness, early detection, and management crucial.

The Importance of Diet in Kidney Health

Diet plays a pivotal role in managing kidney disease and maintaining overall health. For individuals with CKD, dietary modifications can help slow the progression of the disease, manage symptoms, and prevent complications. A kidney-friendly diet typically involves controlling the intake of protein, sodium, potassium, and phosphorus, while ensuring adequate nutrition. This can be particularly challenging, but with the right guidance and delicious recipes, it is entirely achievable.

Why Focus on Women?

While kidney disease affects both men and women, there are specific reasons to focus on a kidney disease diet for women:

1. Hormonal Differences: Women's hormonal fluctuations throughout life stages (menstruation, pregnancy, menopause) can impact kidney function and dietary needs.
2. Bone Health: Women are more prone to osteoporosis, and kidney disease further exacerbates bone health issues due to imbalances in calcium and phosphorus.
3. Heart Health: Women with kidney disease are at higher risk for cardiovascular diseases, necessitating a heart-healthy diet alongside kidney management.
4. Tailored Nutritional Needs: Women have different caloric and nutritional requirements, which should be reflected in a diet plan.

Goals of This Cookbook

The aim of this cookbook is to provide women with kidney disease practical, delicious, and nutritious recipes that cater to their specific health needs. The recipes included are designed to:

1. Support Kidney Function: By managing the intake of key nutrients that affect kidney health.
2. Enhance Overall Well-being: Focusing on balanced nutrition to support other aspects of health.
3. Promote Enjoyment and Satisfaction: Offering a variety of tasty meals that make dietary restrictions easier to adhere to.

What to Expect

In this cookbook, you'll find:

- Educational Content: Each chapter begins with an informative section that explains the dietary principles relevant to kidney disease.
- Practical Tips: Helpful advice on meal planning, grocery shopping, and cooking techniques to support a kidney-friendly diet.
- Diverse Recipes: A wide range of recipes, from breakfast to dinner, snacks to desserts, all designed to be kidney-friendly and delicious.
- Nutritional Information: Each recipe includes detailed nutritional information to help you keep track of your intake of crucial nutrients.

How to Use This Cookbook

This cookbook is designed to be a practical guide and resource. You can read it cover to cover to gain a comprehensive understanding of managing kidney disease through diet, or you can jump to specific sections or recipes that interest you. Each recipe is crafted to be easy to follow, with ingredients that are accessible and methods that are straightforward.

Final Thoughts

Managing kidney disease through diet can seem daunting, but it is a vital part of maintaining health and quality of life. This cookbook aims to empower you with the knowledge and tools you need to make informed dietary choices, while still enjoying delicious and satisfying meals. Remember, you are not alone on this journey—whether you are newly diagnosed or have been living with kidney disease for some time, this cookbook is here to support you every step of the way.

Chapter 2
Understanding

Kidney Disease and Diet

The kidneys play a crucial role in filtering waste products, excess fluids, and toxins from the blood, which are then excreted in the urine. When the kidneys are damaged, these waste products build up in the body, leading to various health complications.

Stages of CKD:

CKD is classified into five stages, based on the glomerular filtration rate (GFR), which measures how well the kidneys are filtering blood:

- Stage 1: Normal or high GFR (90 mL/min or more) but with signs of kidney damage.
- Stage 2: Mild reduction in GFR (60-89 mL/min) with kidney damage.
- Stage 3: Moderate reduction in GFR (30-59 mL/min).
- Stage 4: Severe reduction in GFR (15-29 mL/min).
- Stage 5: Kidney failure (GFR less than 15 mL/min), requiring dialysis or a kidney transplant.

Causes of Kidney Disease

Several factors can lead to the development of CKD, including:

1. Diabetes: High blood sugar levels can damage the blood vessels in the kidneys.

2. High Blood Pressure: Increased pressure can damage the kidney's filtering units.
3. Glomerulonephritis: Inflammation of the kidney's filtering units.
4. Polycystic Kidney Disease: A genetic disorder causing cysts in the kidneys.
5. Urinary Tract Obstructions: Conditions that block the flow of urine.
6. Repeated Kidney Infections: Chronic pyelonephritis can lead to kidney damage.

Symptoms of Kidney Disease

In the early stages, CKD may present no symptoms. As the disease progresses, symptoms may include:

- Fatigue and weakness
- Swelling in the legs, ankles, or feet
- Shortness of breath
- Nausea and vomiting
- Loss of appetite
- Persistent itching
- Changes in urination (frequency, color, and amount)

The Role of Diet in Managing Kidney Disease

Diet is a cornerstone of managing CKD. Proper nutrition can help slow the progression of the disease, manage symptoms, and prevent complications. Key dietary components to consider include:

1. Protein:
    - Why It Matters: Excessive protein intake can put extra strain on the kidneys.

- Recommendation: Limit protein to prevent further damage while ensuring adequate intake for body functions.

2. Sodium:
    - Why It Matters: High sodium intake can lead to high blood pressure and fluid retention.
    - Recommendation: Reduce sodium intake by avoiding processed foods and adding minimal salt during cooking.

3. Potassium:
    - Why It Matters: The kidneys regulate potassium levels, and with CKD, high potassium can lead to heart problems.
    - Recommendation: Monitor and limit high-potassium foods like bananas, oranges, and potatoes.

4. Phosphorus:
    - Why It Matters: High phosphorus levels can weaken bones and cause heart disease.
    - Recommendation: Avoid foods high in phosphorus, such as dairy products, nuts, and certain meats.

5. Fluids:
    - Why It Matters: Managing fluid intake is crucial to avoid fluid overload, which can cause swelling and high blood pressure.
    - Recommendation: Follow a healthcare provider's advice on fluid intake, which varies based on disease stage and symptoms.

Specific Nutritional Needs for Women with Kidney Disease

Women with CKD have unique nutritional needs that must be addressed:

1. Bone Health: Women are at higher risk of osteoporosis, and CKD can exacerbate this risk. Ensuring adequate calcium and vitamin D intake while managing phosphorus levels is vital.
2. Heart Health: Cardiovascular health is closely linked to kidney health, and women with CKD need a diet that supports heart health, including healthy fats and fiber.
3. Reproductive Health: For women of childbearing age, maintaining a balanced diet that supports overall health, including iron and folic acid, is important.

Developing a Kidney-Friendly Diet

Creating a kidney-friendly diet involves balancing various nutrients while considering individual health needs and preferences. Key strategies include:

1. Meal Planning: Plan meals around kidney-friendly foods, incorporating a variety of fruits, vegetables, lean proteins, and whole grains.
2. Reading Labels: Learn to read food labels to identify and avoid high-sodium, high-potassium, and high-phosphorus ingredients.
3. Cooking Methods: Opt for cooking methods that retain nutrients without adding extra sodium or unhealthy fats, such as steaming, grilling, and baking.

Working with Healthcare Professionals

Consulting with a dietitian specialized in kidney disease is highly recommended. They can provide personalized dietary advice, help develop meal plans, and ensure nutritional needs are met while managing CKD. Regular follow-ups with healthcare providers are essential to monitor kidney function and adjust the diet as needed.

Chapter 3
Nutrition Guidelines for Kidney Disease

Protein is vital for body functions, including tissue repair, muscle building, and immune function. However, in CKD, the kidneys struggle to process protein waste, leading to a buildup of urea in the blood. Managing protein intake is essential to reduce the burden on the kidneys while maintaining overall health.

Guidelines:

- Moderate Protein Intake: Typically, 0.6 to 0.8 grams of protein per kilogram of body weight per day is recommended for CKD patients. This amount may vary based on individual needs and disease stage.
- High-Quality Protein Sources: Opt for high-quality proteins that provide essential amino acids, such as lean meats, poultry, fish, eggs, and plant-based proteins like beans and lentils.
- Balance: Distribute protein intake evenly throughout the day to avoid excessive strain on the kidneys.

Sodium Control

Importance of Sodium in CKD:
Sodium regulates blood pressure and fluid balance. In CKD, excess sodium can lead to hypertension, fluid retention, and edema, exacerbating kidney damage.

Guidelines:

- Daily Intake: Limit sodium intake to 1,500 to 2,300 milligrams per day.
- Avoid Processed Foods: Processed foods, canned goods, and fast foods often contain high sodium levels. Choose fresh, whole foods instead.

- Flavor Alternatives: Use herbs, spices, lemon juice, and vinegar to flavor food instead of salt.

Potassium Management

Importance of Potassium in CKD:
Potassium is crucial for nerve and muscle function, including heart rhythm. Impaired kidneys cannot efficiently remove excess potassium, which can lead to hyperkalemia, a potentially life-threatening condition.

Guidelines:

- Monitor Intake: Potassium needs vary; typically, 2,000 to 3,000 milligrams per day is advised, but individual recommendations depend on blood levels.
- Low-Potassium Foods: Choose apples, berries, grapes, cabbage, and cauliflower over high-potassium foods like bananas, oranges, tomatoes, and potatoes.
- Preparation Techniques: Leaching vegetables (soaking in water) before cooking can reduce potassium content.

Phosphorus Control

Importance of Phosphorus in CKD:
Phosphorus is essential for bone health. CKD can cause phosphorus to accumulate, leading to weakened bones and calcification of blood vessels and organs.

Guidelines:

- Daily Intake: Limit phosphorus to 800 to 1,000 milligrams per day.

- Avoid High-Phosphorus Foods: Reduce intake of dairy products, nuts, seeds, whole grains, and certain meats.
- Phosphate Binders: These medications can help reduce phosphorus absorption from foods; consult with a healthcare provider.

Fluid Management

Importance of Fluid in CKD:
Proper fluid balance is vital to prevent dehydration and overhydration, both of which can stress the kidneys and affect overall health.

Guidelines:

- Individual Needs: Fluid needs vary based on disease stage and individual circumstances; follow healthcare provider recommendations.
- Monitor Intake: Track all liquids consumed, including soups, ice cream, and fruits with high water content.
- Symptoms of Imbalance: Watch for signs of overhydration (swelling, shortness of breath) and dehydration (dark urine, dry mouth).

Micronutrient Considerations

Calcium and Vitamin D:

- Bone Health: CKD patients are at risk for bone diseases due to imbalances in calcium and vitamin D.
- Supplements: Supplements may be necessary, but should be taken under medical supervision to avoid complications.

Iron:

- Prevent Anemia: CKD can cause anemia, making iron-rich foods and possibly iron supplements important.
- Sources: Include lean meats, beans, and fortified cereals, but be mindful of phosphorus content in these foods.

Special Considerations for Women

Bone Health:

- Osteoporosis Risk: Women are more prone to osteoporosis, making calcium and vitamin D crucial.
- Balanced Diet: Ensure a diet rich in bone-supporting nutrients while managing phosphorus levels.

Reproductive Health:

- Nutritional Needs: Women of childbearing age should ensure sufficient intake of folic acid, iron, and other vital nutrients.
- Pregnancy: Pregnant women with CKD require specialized dietary plans to support both maternal and fetal health.

Practical Tips for Implementing Kidney-Friendly Diet

1. Meal Planning: Plan meals in advance to ensure they meet nutritional guidelines and dietary restrictions.
2. Cooking Techniques: Use cooking methods that preserve nutrients and flavor without adding sodium or unhealthy fats.
3. Label Reading: Learn to read food labels to identify hidden sources of sodium, potassium, and phosphorus.

4. Portion Control: Manage portion sizes to control nutrient intake effectively.
5. Hydration Management: Track fluid intake diligently, especially if fluid restrictions are in place.

Chapter 4
Meal Planning and Preparation

Effective meal planning is crucial for managing kidney disease. It helps ensure that nutritional needs are met while adhering to dietary restrictions, thereby supporting kidney function and overall health. Proper meal planning also reduces the risk of inadvertently consuming harmful levels of certain nutrients such as sodium, potassium, and phosphorus.

Steps to Effective Meal Planning

1. Understand Nutritional Requirements:
    - Familiarize yourself with the specific dietary needs for kidney disease, including limits on protein, sodium, potassium, phosphorus, and fluid intake.
    - Keep a list of kidney-friendly foods and those to avoid.
2. Plan Balanced Meals:
    - Include a variety of foods to ensure a balanced intake of nutrients.
    - Distribute protein evenly throughout the day to avoid excessive strain on the kidneys.
3. Create a Weekly Menu:

- Plan meals and snacks for the week, taking into account your nutritional goals and dietary restrictions.
  - Ensure each meal includes a balance of protein, carbohydrates, and healthy fats, with controlled portions of high-potassium and high-phosphorus foods.
4. Grocery Shopping:
  - Make a detailed shopping list based on your meal plan.
  - Focus on fresh, whole foods such as fruits, vegetables, lean meats, and whole grains.
  - Avoid processed and convenience foods that often contain high levels of sodium and other additives.

Meal Preparation Tips

1. Batch Cooking:
  - Prepare large quantities of kidney-friendly dishes and portion them out for the week.
  - Freeze individual servings to have ready-made meals that adhere to your dietary needs.
2. Cooking Techniques:
  - Use cooking methods that enhance flavor without adding extra sodium or unhealthy fats, such as grilling, baking, steaming, and stir-frying.
  - Avoid deep frying and excessive use of butter or oils high in saturated fats.
3. Flavoring Food:
  - Use herbs, spices, lemon juice, and vinegar to enhance the flavor of your dishes without adding salt.
  - Experiment with different spice blends to keep meals interesting.
4. Portion Control:

- Use measuring cups and food scales to ensure portion sizes are appropriate.
- Be mindful of serving sizes, especially for protein-rich foods and those high in potassium and phosphorus.

Sample Meal Plan

Day 1:

- Breakfast: Oatmeal with blueberries and a splash of almond milk
- Snack: Sliced apple with a small handful of unsalted almonds
- Lunch: Grilled chicken salad with mixed greens, cucumber, and a lemon vinaigrette
- Snack: Carrot sticks with hummus
- Dinner: Baked salmon with a side of steamed broccoli and quinoa
- Snack: Low-potassium fruit salad (e.g., strawberries, blueberries)

Day 2:

- Breakfast: Scrambled eggs with spinach and a slice of whole grain toast
- Snack: Pear slices with cottage cheese (low-sodium)
- Lunch: Turkey and avocado wrap with lettuce and tomato in a whole grain tortilla
- Snack: Greek yogurt with a sprinkle of cinnamon
- Dinner: Stir-fried tofu with bell peppers, onions, and snap peas served over brown rice
- Snack: Rice cakes with a light spread of peanut butter

Special Considerations for Meal Preparation

1. Leaching Vegetables:
    - For high-potassium vegetables, use the leaching method: peel and soak them in water for at least two hours before cooking, then boil in fresh water to reduce potassium content.
2. Using Low-Sodium Alternatives:
    - Choose low-sodium or sodium-free versions of common ingredients like broths, sauces, and canned goods.
3. Homemade vs. Store-Bought:
    - Whenever possible, prepare meals and snacks at home to have better control over the ingredients and nutrient content.
    - If using store-bought items, read labels carefully and select those that fit within your dietary guidelines.

Managing Fluid Intake

1. Track All Fluids:
    - Keep a log of all fluid intake, including soups, beverages, and foods with high water content.
    - Use smaller cups and sips throughout the day to manage fluid intake without feeling deprived.
2. Flavorful Hydration:
    - Infuse water with slices of lemon, cucumber, or mint to make drinking water more enjoyable without adding excessive fluids.

Preparing for Dining Out

1. Research Menus:

- Look up restaurant menus in advance to find kidney-friendly options.
- Choose dishes that are grilled, baked, or steamed and ask for sauces and dressings on the side.

2. Communicate Dietary Needs:
    - Inform the server about your dietary restrictions and ask for modifications to meet your needs.
    - Don't be afraid to ask for special preparations, such as no added salt.

1.

Chapter 5
Breakfast Recipes

Recipe 1: Blueberry Oatmeal

Ingredients:

- 1/2 cup old-fashioned oats
- 1 cup water
- 1/4 cup fresh or frozen blueberries
- 1/4 cup almond milk (unsweetened)
- 1 tablespoon chia seeds (optional)
- 1 teaspoon honey or maple syrup (optional)
- A pinch of cinnamon

Instructions:

1. In a small pot, bring the water to a boil.
2. Add the oats and reduce the heat to a simmer. Cook for about 5 minutes, stirring occasionally, until the oats are soft.
3. Stir in the blueberries, almond milk, chia seeds (if using), and cinnamon.
4. Cook for an additional 2-3 minutes until the blueberries are warm and the oatmeal reaches your desired consistency.
5. Remove from heat and sweeten with honey or maple syrup if desired.
6. Serve warm and enjoy!

Nutritional Information (per serving):

- Calories: 180
- Protein: 5g
- Sodium: 40mg
- Potassium: 150mg
- Phosphorus: 100mg

Recipe 2: Spinach and Mushroom Egg Scramble

Ingredients:

- 2 large eggs or 1/2 cup egg substitute
- 1/4 cup fresh spinach, chopped
- 1/4 cup mushrooms, sliced
- 1 tablespoon onion, finely chopped
- 1 tablespoon olive oil
- Salt and pepper to taste
- Fresh herbs (optional, for garnish)

Instructions:

1. Heat the olive oil in a non-stick skillet over medium heat.
2. Add the onions and mushrooms and sauté until softened, about 3-4 minutes.
3. Add the spinach and cook until wilted, about 1-2 minutes.
4. In a bowl, whisk the eggs with a pinch of salt and pepper.
5. Pour the eggs into the skillet with the vegetables and cook, stirring gently, until the eggs are fully cooked but still moist.
6. Serve immediately, garnished with fresh herbs if desired.

Nutritional Information (per serving):

- Calories: 180
- Protein: 12g
- Sodium: 140mg
- Potassium: 250mg
- Phosphorus: 200mg

Recipe 3: Apple Cinnamon Quinoa

Ingredients:

- 1/2 cup quinoa
- 1 cup water
- 1/2 apple, chopped
- 1/4 teaspoon cinnamon
- 1 teaspoon honey or maple syrup (optional)
- 1/4 cup almond milk (unsweetened)
- 1 tablespoon chopped walnuts (optional)

Instructions:

1. Rinse the quinoa under cold water.
2. In a small pot, bring the water to a boil. Add the quinoa, reduce the heat to low, and cover. Cook for about 15 minutes or until the water is absorbed and the quinoa is fluffy.
3. Stir in the chopped apple, cinnamon, and almond milk. Cook for another 2-3 minutes until the apple is slightly softened.
4. Remove from heat and sweeten with honey or maple syrup if desired.
5. Sprinkle with chopped walnuts if using, and serve warm.

Nutritional Information (per serving):

- Calories: 220
- Protein: 6g
- Sodium: 10mg
- Potassium: 200mg
- Phosphorus: 140mg

Recipe 4: Greek Yogurt with Berries and Honey

Ingredients:

- 1/2 cup plain Greek yogurt (low-fat or non-fat)
- 1/4 cup mixed berries (strawberries, blueberries, raspberries)
- 1 teaspoon honey
- 1 tablespoon chia seeds (optional)

Instructions:

1. In a bowl, mix the Greek yogurt with the chia seeds (if using).
2. Top with mixed berries.
3. Drizzle with honey.
4. Serve immediately and enjoy!

Nutritional Information (per serving):

- Calories: 150
- Protein: 10g
- Sodium: 60mg
- Potassium: 200mg
- Phosphorus: 150mg

Recipe 5: Avocado and Tomato Toast

Ingredients:

- 1 slice whole grain bread, toasted
- 1/4 ripe avocado
- 1 small tomato, sliced
- A squeeze of lemon juice
- Salt and pepper to taste

Instructions:

1. Toast the whole grain bread to your desired crispiness.
2. In a small bowl, mash the avocado with a fork and mix
    in a squeeze of lemon juice, salt, and pepper.
3. Spread the avocado mixture onto the toasted bread.
4. Top with sliced tomato.
5. Serve immediately and enjoy!

Nutritional Information (per serving):

- Calories: 200
- Protein: 5g
- Sodium: 150mg
- Potassium: 350mg
- Phosphorus: 100mg

Chapter 6
Lunch Recipes

Recipe 1: Grilled Chicken and Quinoa Salad

Ingredients:

- 1/2 cup quinoa
- 1 cup water
- 1 small chicken breast, grilled and sliced
- 1/2 cup cherry tomatoes, halved
- 1/2 cucumber, diced
- 1/4 cup red bell pepper, diced
- 1 tablespoon olive oil
- 1 tablespoon lemon juice
- 1 tablespoon fresh parsley, chopped

- Salt and pepper to taste

Instructions:

1. Rinse the quinoa under cold water. In a small pot, bring the water to a boil, then add the quinoa. Reduce heat, cover, and simmer for about 15 minutes, or until the water is absorbed and the quinoa is fluffy. Let it cool.
2. In a large bowl, combine the cooled quinoa, grilled chicken, cherry tomatoes, cucumber, and red bell pepper.
3. In a small bowl, whisk together the olive oil, lemon juice, parsley, salt, and pepper.
4. Pour the dressing over the quinoa salad and toss to combine.
5. Serve chilled or at room temperature.

Nutritional Information (per serving):

- Calories: 350
- Protein: 25g
- Sodium: 150mg

- Potassium: 400mg

- Phosphorus: 250mg

Recipe 2: Turkey and Avocado Wrap

Ingredients:

- 1 whole grain tortilla

- 2-3 slices of low-sodium turkey breast

- 1/4 ripe avocado, sliced

- 1/2 cup mixed greens (lettuce, spinach)

- 1/4 cup shredded carrots

- 1 tablespoon hummus (optional)

- A squeeze of lemon juice

- Salt and pepper to taste

Instructions:

1. Lay the tortilla flat and spread a thin layer of hummus (if using).

2. Layer the turkey slices, avocado, mixed greens, and shredded carrots on the tortilla.

3. Squeeze a bit of lemon juice over the fillings and
    season with salt and pepper.

4. Roll up the tortilla tightly, tucking in the sides as you go.

5. Cut the wrap in half and serve immediately.

Nutritional Information (per serving):

- Calories: 300

- Protein: 18g

- Sodium: 250mg

- Potassium: 450mg

- Phosphorus: 180mg

Recipe 3: Veggie Stir-Fry with Tofu

Ingredients:

- 1/2 block firm tofu, cubed

- 1 tablespoon olive oil

- 1 cup broccoli florets

- 1/2 cup bell pepper, sliced

- 1/2 cup snow peas

- 1 small carrot, julienned

- 2 tablespoons low-sodium soy sauce

- 1 tablespoon rice vinegar

- 1 teaspoon fresh ginger, grated

- 1 garlic clove, minced

- Cooked brown rice (optional, for serving)

Instructions:

1. Heat the olive oil in a large skillet over medium-high heat. Add the tofu cubes and cook until golden brown on all sides. Remove from the skillet and set aside.

2. In the same skillet, add the broccoli, bell pepper, snow peas, and carrot. Stir-fry for 5-7 minutes until the vegetables are tender-crisp.

3. In a small bowl, whisk together the soy sauce, rice vinegar, ginger, and garlic.

4. Return the tofu to the skillet and pour the sauce over the tofu and vegetables. Stir to coat everything evenly.

5. Cook for an additional 2-3 minutes until heated through.

6. Serve the stir-fry over cooked brown rice if desired.

Nutritional Information (per serving):

- Calories: 280

- Protein: 15g

- Sodium: 320mg

- Potassium: 450mg

- Phosphorus: 200mg

Recipe 4: Lentil and Vegetable Soup

Ingredients:

- 1/2 cup dried lentils, rinsed

- 1 small onion, diced

- 1 celery stalk, diced

- 1 carrot, diced

- 1 garlic clove, minced

- 1 tablespoon olive oil

- 4 cups low-sodium vegetable broth

- 1 can (14.5 ounces) diced tomatoes, no salt added

- 1 teaspoon dried thyme

- 1 teaspoon dried basil

- 1 bay leaf

- Salt and pepper to taste

- Fresh parsley, chopped (optional, for garnish)

Instructions:

1. In a large pot, heat the olive oil over medium heat. Add the onion, celery, carrot, and garlic. Sauté until the vegetables are softened, about 5 minutes.

2. Add the lentils, vegetable broth, diced tomatoes, thyme, basil, bay leaf, salt, and pepper. Bring to a boil.

3. Reduce heat and simmer for about 30 minutes, or until the lentils are tender.

4. Remove the bay leaf before serving.

5. Garnish with fresh parsley if desired and serve hot.

Nutritional Information (per serving):

- Calories: 250

- Protein: 12g

- Sodium: 150mg

- Potassium: 600mg

- Phosphorus: 200mg

Recipe 5: Chicken and Zucchini Pasta

Ingredients:

- 1 small chicken breast, cooked and sliced

- 1 medium zucchini, spiralized into noodles (zoodles)

- 1 cup cherry tomatoes, halved

- 1 tablespoon olive oil

- 1 garlic clove, minced

- 1 tablespoon fresh basil, chopped

- Salt and pepper to taste

- Grated Parmesan cheese (optional, for garnish)

Instructions:

1. Heat the olive oil in a large skillet over medium heat. Add the garlic and sauté until fragrant, about 1 minute.

2. Add the cherry tomatoes and cook for 3-4 minutes until they start to soften.

3. Add the zucchini noodles and cooked chicken to the skillet. Cook for an additional 3-4 minutes until the zucchini is tender.

4. Season with salt, pepper, and fresh basil.

5. Serve immediately, topped with grated Parmesan cheese if desired.

Nutritional Information (per serving):

- Calories: 270
- Protein: 25g
- Sodium: 140mg
- Potassium: 800mg
- Phosphorus: 250mg

Chapter 7
Dinner Recipes

Recipe 1: Baked Salmon with Asparagus

Ingredients:

- 1 salmon fillet (4-6 ounces)
- 1 tablespoon olive oil
- 1 garlic clove, minced
- 1 lemon, sliced
- 1 bunch asparagus, trimmed
- 1 tablespoon fresh dill, chopped
- Salt and pepper to taste

Instructions:

1. Preheat the oven to 375°F (190°C).
2. Place the salmon fillet on a baking sheet lined with parchment paper. Drizzle with olive oil and sprinkle with minced garlic, salt, and pepper.

3. Arrange lemon slices on top of the salmon.
4. On the same baking sheet, place the asparagus and drizzle with a bit more olive oil, salt, and pepper.
5. Bake for 15-20 minutes, until the salmon is cooked through and flakes easily with a fork and the asparagus is tender.
6. Sprinkle fresh dill over the salmon before serving.

Nutritional Information (per serving):

- Calories: 350
- Protein: 28g
- Sodium: 100mg
- Potassium: 600mg
- Phosphorus: 250mg

Recipe 2: Herb-Roasted Chicken with Vegetables

Ingredients:

- 1 small chicken breast, bone-in and skin-on
- 1 tablespoon olive oil
- 1 teaspoon dried thyme
- 1 teaspoon dried rosemary
- 1 garlic clove, minced
- 1 carrot, chopped
- 1 potato, chopped
- 1/2 cup green beans, trimmed
- Salt and pepper to taste

Instructions:

1. Preheat the oven to 375°F (190°C).
2. In a small bowl, mix the olive oil, thyme, rosemary, garlic, salt, and pepper.

3. Rub the chicken breast with the herb mixture and place it in a roasting pan.
4. Add the chopped carrot, potato, and green beans to the pan, tossing them in any remaining herb mixture.
5. Roast for about 45 minutes, or until the chicken is cooked through and the vegetables are tender.
6. Serve hot.

Nutritional Information (per serving):

- Calories: 400
- Protein: 30g
- Sodium: 200mg
- Potassium: 700mg
- Phosphorus: 280mg

Recipe 3: Stuffed Bell Peppers

Ingredients:

- 2 large bell peppers, halved and seeds removed
- 1/2 cup quinoa, cooked
- 1/2 cup black beans, rinsed and drained
- 1/2 cup corn kernels (fresh or frozen)
- 1 small tomato, diced
- 1 tablespoon olive oil
- 1 teaspoon cumin
- 1 teaspoon chili powder
- 1/4 cup shredded cheddar cheese (optional)
- Salt and pepper to taste
- Fresh cilantro, chopped (optional, for garnish)

Instructions:

1. Preheat the oven to 375°F (190°C).

2. In a large bowl, combine the cooked quinoa, black beans, corn, diced tomato, olive oil, cumin, chili powder, salt, and pepper.
3. Stuff the bell pepper halves with the quinoa mixture and place them in a baking dish.
4. Cover the dish with foil and bake for 25-30 minutes, until the peppers are tender.
5. If using, sprinkle shredded cheddar cheese on top of the peppers and bake uncovered for an additional 5 minutes, until the cheese is melted.
6. Garnish with fresh cilantro before serving.

Nutritional Information (per serving):

- Calories: 250
- Protein: 8g
- Sodium: 150mg
- Potassium: 500mg
- Phosphorus: 150mg

Recipe 4: Turkey Meatballs with Zucchini Noodles

Ingredients:

- 1/2 pound ground turkey
- 1/4 cup breadcrumbs (low-sodium)
- 1 egg, beaten
- 1 garlic clove, minced
- 1 tablespoon fresh parsley, chopped
- 1 tablespoon olive oil
- 2 medium zucchinis, spiralized into noodles (zoodles)
- 1 cup marinara sauce (low-sodium)
- Salt and pepper to taste

Instructions:

1. In a bowl, combine the ground turkey, breadcrumbs, egg, garlic, parsley, salt, and pepper. Mix well and form into small meatballs.
2. Heat the olive oil in a large skillet over medium heat. Add the meatballs and cook until browned on all sides and cooked through, about 10-15 minutes. Remove from the skillet and set aside.
3. In the same skillet, add the zucchini noodles and sauté for 2-3 minutes until just tender.
4. Add the marinara sauce and meatballs back to the skillet, stirring to coat everything evenly with the sauce. Cook for an additional 2-3 minutes until heated through.
5. Serve immediately.

Nutritional Information (per serving):

- Calories: 300
- Protein: 22g
- Sodium: 200mg
- Potassium: 550mg
- Phosphorus: 220mg

Recipe 5: Vegetable Stir-Fry with Shrimp

Ingredients:

- 1/2 pound shrimp, peeled and deveined
- 1 tablespoon olive oil
- 1 cup broccoli florets
- 1/2 cup bell pepper, sliced
- 1/2 cup snow peas
- 1 small carrot, julienned
- 2 tablespoons low-sodium soy sauce
- 1 tablespoon rice vinegar
- 1 teaspoon fresh ginger, grated
- 1 garlic clove, minced

- Cooked brown rice (optional, for serving)

Instructions:

1. Heat the olive oil in a large skillet or wok over medium-high heat. Add the shrimp and cook until pink and opaque, about 2-3 minutes per side. Remove from the skillet and set aside.
2. In the same skillet, add the broccoli, bell pepper, snow peas, and carrot. Stir-fry for 5-7 minutes until the vegetables are tender-crisp.
3. In a small bowl, whisk together the soy sauce, rice vinegar, ginger, and garlic.
4. Return the shrimp to the skillet and pour the sauce over the shrimp and vegetables. Stir to coat everything evenly.
5. Cook for an additional 2-3 minutes until heated through.
6. Serve the stir-fry over cooked brown rice if desired.

Nutritional Information (per serving):

- Calories: 250
- Protein: 22g
- Sodium: 300mg
- Potassium: 450mg
- Phosphorus: 200mg

Chapter 8
Snacks and Desserts

Snack 1: Greek Yogurt Parfait

Ingredients:

- 1/2 cup plain Greek yogurt (low-fat or non-fat)
- 1/4 cup mixed berries (strawberries, blueberries, raspberries)
- 1 tablespoon chopped nuts (almonds, walnuts)
- 1 teaspoon honey (optional)

Instructions:

1. In a small bowl or glass, layer the Greek yogurt, mixed berries, and chopped nuts.
2. Drizzle with honey if desired.
3. Serve immediately.

Nutritional Information (per serving):

- Calories: 150
- Protein: 10g
- Sodium: 60mg
- Potassium: 200mg
- Phosphorus: 150mg

Snack 2: Veggie Sticks with Hummus

Ingredients:

- Assorted vegetable sticks (carrots, cucumber, bell peppers)
- 2 tablespoons hummus (low-sodium)

Instructions:

1. Wash and cut assorted vegetables into sticks.
2. Serve with hummus for dipping.

Nutritional Information (per serving):

- Calories: 100
- Protein: 4g
- Sodium: 100mg
- Potassium: 250mg
- Phosphorus: 80mg

Snack 3: Rice Cakes with Nut Butter

Ingredients:

- 2 rice cakes (unsalted)
- 2 tablespoons nut butter (almond, peanut)

Instructions:

1. Spread nut butter evenly on rice cakes.
2. Serve as is or top with sliced fruit like banana or apple.

Nutritional Information (per serving):

- Calories: 200
- Protein: 6g
- Sodium: 0mg
- Potassium: 150mg
- Phosphorus: 100mg

Dessert Ideas:

Dessert 1: Berry Smoothie

Ingredients:

- 1/2 cup mixed berries (strawberries, blueberries, raspberries)
- 1/2 cup plain Greek yogurt (low-fat or non-fat)
- 1/4 cup almond milk (unsweetened)
- 1 teaspoon honey (optional)
- Ice cubes

Instructions:

1. Combine mixed berries, Greek yogurt, almond milk, and honey in a blender.
2. Add ice cubes as desired for thickness.
3. Blend until smooth and creamy.
4. Pour into a glass and serve immediately.

Nutritional Information (per serving):

- Calories: 150
- Protein: 10g
- Sodium: 60mg

- Potassium: 200mg
- Phosphorus: 150mg

Dessert 2: Baked Apples with Cinnamon

Ingredients:

- 2 apples (Granny Smith or Fuji)
- 1 teaspoon cinnamon
- 1 tablespoon chopped nuts (almonds, walnuts)
- 1 teaspoon honey (optional)

Instructions:

1. Preheat the oven to 375°F (190°C).
2. Core the apples and slice off the tops.
3. Sprinkle cinnamon inside each apple and on top.
4. Place the apples in a baking dish and bake for 20-25 minutes until tender.
5. Remove from oven and sprinkle with chopped nuts and drizzle with honey if desired.
6. Serve warm.

Nutritional Information (per serving):

- Calories: 150
- Protein: 2g
- Sodium: 0mg
- Potassium: 200mg
- Phosphorus: 50mg

Dessert 3: Frozen Banana Bites

Ingredients:

- 2 bananas, peeled and cut into slices
- 1/4 cup dark chocolate chips
- 1 tablespoon coconut oil
- Chopped nuts (optional)

Instructions:

1. Place banana slices on a parchment-lined baking sheet.
2. In a microwave-safe bowl, melt dark chocolate chips and coconut oil together in 30-second intervals until smooth.
3. Dip each banana slice halfway into the melted chocolate and place back on the baking sheet.
4. Sprinkle with chopped nuts if desired.
5. Place in the freezer for 1-2 hours until chocolate is set.
6. Serve chilled.

Nutritional Information (per serving):

- Calories: 150
- Protein: 2g
- Sodium: 0mg
- Potassium: 200mg
- Phosphorus: 50mg

Chapter 9
Beverages

Beverage 1: Infused Water

Ingredients:

- Water
- Sliced fruits (lemon, lime, orange, berries)
- Fresh herbs (mint, basil)

Instructions:

1. Fill a pitcher with water.
2. Add sliced fruits and fresh herbs.
3. Refrigerate for at least 2 hours to allow flavors to infuse.
4. Serve chilled over ice.

Benefits:

- Hydrating without added sugars or artificial flavors.
- Provides a refreshing and flavorful alternative to plain water.
- Helps meet daily fluid intake goals.

Beverage 2: Herbal Tea

Ingredients:

- Herbal tea bags (chamomile, peppermint, rooibos)
- Hot water

Instructions:

1. Place herbal tea bag in a cup.
2. Pour hot water over the tea bag.
3. Steep for 5-7 minutes.
4. Remove the tea bag and enjoy.

Benefits:

- Naturally caffeine-free, making it suitable for any time of day.
- May have calming or soothing effects, depending on the herbs used.
- Helps increase fluid intake without added sugars or calories.

Beverage 3: Green Smoothie

Ingredients:

- 1 cup fresh spinach or kale
- 1/2 ripe banana
- 1/2 cup frozen mixed berries
- 1/2 cup plain Greek yogurt (low-fat or non-fat)
- 1/4 cup almond milk (unsweetened)
- Ice cubes (optional)

Instructions:

1. Combine spinach or kale, banana, berries, Greek yogurt, and almond milk in a blender.
2. Blend until smooth and creamy.
3. Add ice cubes if desired for a colder texture.
4. Pour into a glass and serve immediately.

Benefits:

- Provides a nutrient-rich beverage with vitamins and antioxidants from leafy greens and fruits.
- Offers a creamy texture without added sugars or dairy alternatives.
- Supports hydration while contributing to daily fruit and vegetable intake.

Beverage 4: Coconut Water

Ingredients:

- Coconut water (unsweetened)

Instructions:

1. Pour coconut water into a glass.
2. Serve chilled over ice if desired.

Benefits:

- Naturally rich in electrolytes such as potassium and magnesium, which are important for kidney health.
- Provides hydration without added sugars or artificial additives.
- Offers a refreshing and tropical flavor profile.

Beverage 5: Sparkling Water with Lemon or Lime

Ingredients:

- Sparkling water (unsweetened)
- Sliced lemon or lime

Instructions:

1. Pour sparkling water into a glass.
2. Add sliced lemon or lime for flavor.
3. Serve chilled over ice if desired.

Benefits:

- Provides a bubbly and refreshing beverage option without added sugars or calories.
- Enhances hydration with a hint of citrus flavor.
- Satisfies carbonated beverage cravings without the negative effects of soda.

Chapter 10 Navigating a kidney disease diet Lifestyle (Conclusion)

Grocery Shopping Guide for Kidney-Friendly Eating

Navigating the grocery store can be overwhelming, especially when following a kidney-friendly diet. This chapter provides practical tips and strategies for making informed choices and selecting the right foods to support kidney health.

Understanding Food Labels:

- Sodium Content: Look for products labeled "low sodium" or "no added salt." Compare sodium content between similar products and choose the one with the lowest sodium content per serving.

- Potassium and Phosphorus: While these nutrients may not always be listed on nutrition labels, it's essential to be mindful of foods naturally high in potassium and phosphorus. Fresh fruits and vegetables are generally lower in these minerals compared to processed and packaged foods.

- Ingredient Lists: Check for hidden sources of sodium, potassium, and phosphorus in ingredient lists. Ingredients like monosodium glutamate (MSG), potassium chloride, and phosphoric acid indicate the presence of these minerals.

Shopping Strategies:

- Stick to the Perimeter: Fresh produce, lean proteins, and dairy products are typically located around the perimeter of the store. Focus on filling your cart with these kidney-friendly options.

- Choose Fresh and Frozen: Opt for fresh or frozen fruits and vegetables over canned varieties, as they tend to have lower sodium content. Look for unsweetened frozen fruits and vegetables without added sauces or seasonings.

- Select Lean Proteins: Choose lean cuts of meat, poultry, and fish. Trim visible fat and skin from meats to reduce saturated fat intake. Consider incorporating plant-based protein sources such as beans, lentils, and tofu.

- Read Labels Carefully: Pay attention to serving sizes and nutrient content on food labels. Even products marketed as "healthy" or "natural" may contain high levels of sodium, potassium, or phosphorus.

Budget-Friendly Tips:

- Buy in Bulk: Purchase staples like rice, beans, and whole grains in bulk to save money. Store them in airtight containers to maintain freshness.

- Shop Seasonally: Take advantage of seasonal produce, which is often more affordable and at its peak freshness. Consider buying extra and freezing or preserving fruits and vegetables for later use.

- Compare Prices: Compare prices between brands and store brands versus name brands. Look for sales, discounts, and coupons to maximize savings without sacrificing quality.

Stocking a Kidney-Friendly Pantry:

- Whole Grains: Keep a variety of whole grains on hand, such as brown rice, quinoa, oats, and whole wheat pasta.

- Canned Goods: Choose low-sodium or no-salt-added canned beans, tomatoes, and vegetables. Rinse canned beans and vegetables under cold water before using to reduce sodium content.
- Healthy Fats: Stock up on heart-healthy fats like olive oil, avocado oil, and nuts. Use these in cooking and as toppings for salads and snacks.

- Herbs and Spices: Build a collection of herbs, spices, and seasonings to add flavor to dishes without relying on salt. Experiment with garlic, onion powder, oregano, basil, and lemon zest.

Managing Special Dietary Needs and Restrictions

Living with kidney disease often involves managing multiple dietary needs and restrictions, especially if you have other health conditions such as diabetes, hypertension, or food allergies. This chapter provides guidance on navigating these complexities to maintain a healthy and balanced diet.

Understanding Common Dietary Restrictions:

- Diabetes: If you have diabetes along with kidney disease, you'll need to manage your carbohydrate intake to control blood sugar levels. Focus on choosing complex carbohydrates like whole grains, fruits, and vegetables, and monitor portion sizes to avoid spikes in blood sugar.

- Hypertension: High blood pressure is a common complication of kidney disease. Limiting sodium intake is crucial for managing hypertension. Choose low-sodium or no-salt-added foods, and avoid processed and packaged foods, which often contain high levels of sodium.

- Food Allergies: If you have food allergies or intolerances, such as gluten intolerance or lactose intolerance, it's essential to identify and avoid trigger foods. Look for alternative options that meet your dietary needs without compromising kidney health.

Adapting Kidney-Friendly Recipes:

- Low-Carb Modifications: If you're following a low-carbohydrate diet for diabetes management, you can adapt kidney-friendly recipes by choosing lower-carb options for grains and starchy vegetables. Substitute cauliflower rice for regular rice or zucchini noodles for pasta.

- Gluten-Free Options: For individuals with gluten intolerance or celiac disease, opt for gluten-free grains like quinoa, rice, and buckwheat. Look for gluten-free versions of products like pasta and bread or use alternatives like corn tortillas or lettuce wraps.

- Dairy-Free Alternatives: If you're lactose intolerant or following a dairy-free diet, choose non-dairy alternatives such as almond milk, coconut milk, or soy milk. Use dairy-free yogurt and cheese substitutes in recipes that call for dairy products.

Managing Medications and Supplements:

- Medication Interactions: Some medications prescribed for kidney disease management may interact with certain foods or supplements. Consult with your healthcare provider or pharmacist to understand potential interactions and adjust your diet or medication regimen accordingly.

- Nutritional Supplements: Depending on your specific nutritional needs, your healthcare provider may recommend supplements such as vitamin D, iron, or erythropoietin-stimulating agents (ESAs). Follow your healthcare provider's guidance on supplement use and dosage to avoid complications.

Seeking Professional Support:

- Consult a Dietitian: A registered dietitian can provide personalized nutrition counseling and help you develop a meal plan that meets your individual dietary needs and restrictions. They can also offer guidance on managing complex dietary considerations and navigating food choices.

- Collaborate with Healthcare Providers: Work closely with your healthcare team, including your nephrologist, primary care physician, and specialists, to coordinate care and address any concerns related to managing multiple health conditions.

Exercise and Physical Activity for Kidney Health

Physical activity plays a vital role in supporting kidney health and overall well-being for individuals with kidney disease. This chapter provides guidance on the benefits of exercise, safe and effective exercise routines, and strategies for incorporating physical activity into daily life.

Understanding the Benefits of Exercise:

- Improved Cardiovascular Health: Regular exercise helps lower blood pressure, improve cholesterol levels, and reduce the risk of cardiovascular disease, which is common among individuals with kidney disease.

- Enhanced Kidney Function: Physical activity promotes better blood flow to the kidneys, which can help improve kidney function and reduce the risk of complications associated with kidney disease.

- Weight Management: Exercise can aid in weight management by burning calories and building lean muscle mass, which is important for individuals with kidney disease who may be at risk of obesity or overweight.

- Mood Enhancement: Physical activity releases endorphins, chemicals in the brain that promote feelings of happiness and well-being, helping to reduce stress, anxiety, and depression commonly experienced by individuals with kidney disease.

Safe and Effective Exercise Routines:

- Consult with Healthcare Providers: Before starting any exercise program, consult with your healthcare provider, particularly if you have advanced kidney disease or other health conditions. They can provide guidance on appropriate exercise intensity, duration, and frequency based on your individual health status.

- Choose Low-Impact Activities: Opt for low-impact exercises that are gentle on the joints and kidneys, such as walking, swimming, cycling, and tai chi. These activities provide cardiovascular benefits without placing undue stress on the kidneys.

- Gradually Increase Intensity: Start with light-intensity exercise and gradually increase the intensity and duration as your fitness level improves. Listen to your body and avoid pushing yourself too hard, especially if you're just starting out or have limited mobility.

- Incorporate Strength Training: Include strength training exercises in your routine to build muscle strength and improve bone health. Use light weights or resistance bands and focus on performing exercises that target major muscle groups, such as squats, lunges, and bicep curls.

Strategies for Incorporating Physical Activity:

- Set Realistic Goals: Establish achievable fitness goals based on your current fitness level, health status, and personal preferences. Start with small, manageable goals and gradually increase the challenge over time.
- Schedule Regular Workouts: Schedule regular exercise sessions into your weekly routine, just like you would any other important appointment. Aim for at least 30 minutes of moderate-intensity exercise on most days of the week.
- Find Activities You Enjoy: Choose activities that you enjoy and that fit your interests and lifestyle. Whether it's dancing, gardening, or playing a sport, finding

activities that you love will make exercise feel less like a chore and more like a rewarding experience.

- Stay Consistent: Consistency is key to reaping the benefits of exercise for kidney health. Even on days when you don't feel motivated, aim to do some form of physical activity, even if it's just a short walk or gentle stretching routine.

Safety Precautions:

- Stay Hydrated: Drink plenty of water before, during, and after exercise to stay hydrated, especially if you have kidney disease and are at risk of dehydration.
- Monitor Symptoms: Pay attention to how your body feels during and after exercise. If you experience any unusual symptoms such as dizziness, chest pain, or extreme fatigue, stop exercising and consult with your healthcare provider.
- Avoid Overexertion: Be mindful not to overexert yourself, especially if you have kidney disease or other health conditions. Take breaks as needed and listen to your body's cues to avoid pushing yourself too hard.
- Warm Up and Cool Down: Always start your workouts with a gentle warm-up to prepare your muscles and joints for exercise, and finish with a cool-down to gradually lower your heart rate and prevent muscle soreness.

www.ingramcontent.com/pod-product-compliance
Lightning Source LLC
Chambersburg PA
CBHW051701250726
48653CB00007B/2791